The Isometric Workout Routine For Everyone

By Anthony Anholt

Copyright © 2012 By Anthony Anholt

Illustrated By Jonathan Fesmire

https://www.elance.com/s/jfesmire/

http://jonfesmire.com/

Disclaimer

The exercises and advice contained within this course may be too strenuous or dangerous for some people, and the reader(s) should consult a physician before engaging in them. The author and publisher of this course are not responsible in any manner whatsoever for any injury which may occur through reading and following the instructions herein.

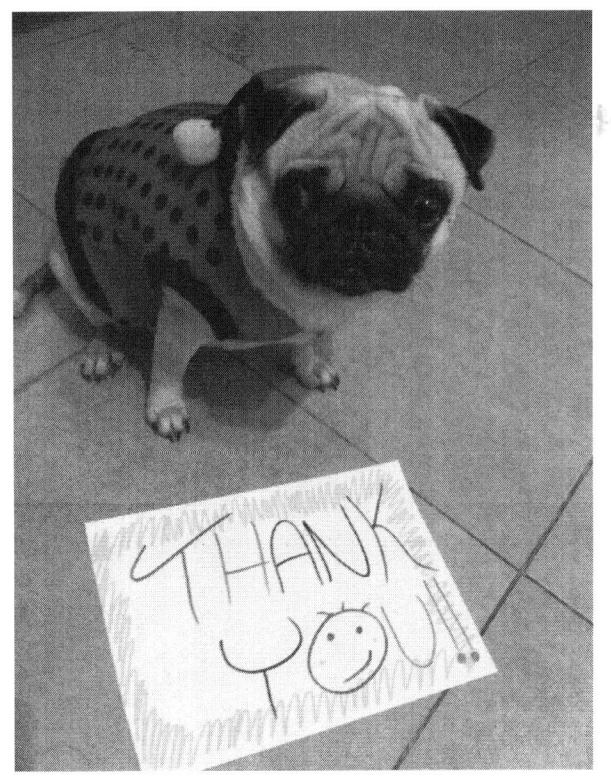

Thank-you for purchasing my book. Please REVIEW my book on Amazon. I appreciate your feedback so that I can make the next version even better. Thank-you so much!

Table Of Contents

How Isometric Exercises Can Benefit You	5
What Are Isometric Exercises?	6
How To Perform An Isometric Contraction	8
More Tips On Performing Isometric Exercises	9
How To Perform This Isometric Workout	11
Abdominal Exercises	12
Isometric Stomach Flattener	12
Oblique Door Press	14
Exercises For The Neck	16
Reverse Neck Contraction	16
Forward Neck Contraction	18
Side Neck Contraction	20
Exercises For The Back	22
Trapezius Contraction	22
The Isometric Row	24
Sitting Isometric Pull	26
Isometric Wall Press	28
Isometric Broom Pull	30
Isometric Superman	32
Shoulder Exercises	34
Isometric Shoulder Press	34
Front Shoulder Raise	36

Side Shoulder Raise	38
Rear Shoulder Pull	40
Isometric Arm Exercises	42
Biceps Curl	42
Triceps Press Down	44
Isometric Cross Arm Contraction	46
Chest Exercises	48
Isometric Pec Builder (Push)	48
Isometric Pec Builder (Pull)	50
Isometric Pushup	52
Leg Exercises	54
Wall Squat	54
Leg Curl	56
Front Thigh Exercise	58
Inner Thigh Exercise	60
Outer Thigh Exercise	62
The Isometric Atlas	64
About The Author	66
One Last Thing	67

Isometric Exercise Can Benefit You

I know a person who owns a Porsche sports car. It's his baby and he cares for it almost as if it were one of his children. He spends a LOT of money on regular tune-ups (I've learned it costs a lot more to maintain a fancy sports car than say, a Honda Civic) and when he parks his car he covers it with a tarp. In addition to this he makes sure he drives it regularly, even if he has nowhere to go. The reason he does this is that he knows that a sports car is meant to be used. If you want to keep a Porsche in tiptop condition, you have to let it do what it was designed to do, which is to be driven (sometimes quite fast).

Most of us will never own a Porsche, and yet we all possess a machine that makes the Porsche pale in comparison. That machine is your body. More wondrous than a sports car and more fine-tuned than a Swiss watch, your body is an amazing machine. What's more, it needs to be cared for and used as well. Your body is more amazing than any sports car. Shouldn't you treat it like one?

However, whereas cars require maintenance to stay in top form, human beings require exercise. In the not so distant past people used to get exercise, whether they wanted it or not, by performing hard, difficult labor. In the modern world though this just isn't the case. Most of us don't work on farms anymore, and even those that do rely on machines. Although the times have changed, our bodies haven't. In order to stay in tiptop condition they still need to move and be worked. Most of us know this, but the time pressures put on us by modern society makes following any kind of exercise program difficult. This is why following a system of isometrics can be so valuable to you as isometrics, unique among forms of exercise, can be done quickly and easily, anywhere at anytime.

What Are Isometric Exercises?

Isometric training involves working your muscles without actually moving them. It utilizes a principle known as the isometric contraction to accomplish this. Here's the science behind this idea.

Your muscles are made up of thousands of individual muscle fibers. It is these fibers that contract when you move a limb like your arm. Traditional forms of exercise, such as weight lifting, build muscle by progressively tiring out these fibers to a point of failure. As an example, let's say you are doing a bicep curl with a dumbbell. In order to move the dumbbell through the range of motion your brain activates muscle fibers to contract so that your arm can curl the weight. As you curl the dumbbell multiple times you will tire out these muscle fibers, forcing your brain to activate other, "fresher" fibers. The idea behind weightlifting is that you keep doing this until you have exhausted all of the muscle fibers in question. This works, but it can be time consuming. Wouldn't it be great if you could work all of those same muscle fibers at once?

This is essentially the idea behind isometric exercise. To demonstrate this concept imagine how your brain reacts if you start pressing against an immovable object, like a brick wall. Your brain will very quickly activate all the muscle fibers at its disposal in an (likely futile) attempt to move that wall. This process, by which all of the muscle fibers are used without actually moving, is known as an isometric contraction. The result is that while it takes many sets and reps to work all the muscle fibers lifting weights, you can hit them all in seconds using isometrics.

If the above confuses you, look at it this way. In order to pick up something light, like a paper cup, your brain only needs to activate a few muscle fibers. If you pick up something heavier, such as a barbell, your brain will activate more, but only enough to actually lift the barbell. Your brain will always only activate the muscle fibers it needs to accomplish a task. When it is faced with a task that it cannot accomplish, like pushing over a building, it will still try. This is why all the muscle fibers will get activated almost instantaneously. This is the principle behind the isometric contraction and is why isometrics can be so effective and yet save you so much time.

How To Perform An Isometric Contraction

This book is a series of exercises based on this principle. However, instead of pushing against walls we will, for the most part, be using self-resistance. Before we get to the exercises though I need to explain the proper breathing procedure to follow in order to perform these exercises. The key point is that at no time when performing these exercises should you ever hold your breath. Isometrics are easy to do, but they are not easy. When you hold your breath it is possible to raise your blood pressure to dangerous levels. This could result in suffering a fainting episode or worse. Never do this! Instead, follow the breathing procedure listed below in order to perform these exercises safely and effectively at all times.

1. Breathe in through your nose for 3 seconds are you begin to build tension in your muscles. During this 3-second interval you should be building the muscle tension from nothing to the maximum amount you're capable of exerting.
2. When you reach the point of maximum tension after 3 seconds you will want to hold this contraction for 7 seconds. As you do so breathe out through your mouth by making a "sssssss" sound. This is accomplished by placing your tongue on the roof of your mouth as you

8

3. powerfully force air through your almost clenched teeth.
3. After 7 seconds has passed begin to relax the isometric contraction over a period of 3 seconds. While you do this make sure you breathe in through your nose.

And that's really all there is to it. Breathe in though your nose for 3 seconds as you build tension, exhale for 7 seconds as you hold the contraction, and then breathe in again through your nose. If you follow this procedure you will be able to perform these exercises safely and effectively.

More Tips On Performing Isometric Exercises

- When starting out you may want to use a clock with a second hand to make sure you are accurately counting time during the breathing procedure. If you don't have access to an accurate timepiece you can always count "One thousand one, one thousand two" in your head.
- Remember; NEVER AT ANYTIME HOLD YOUR BREATH. (I know I'm repeating myself, but I can't stress this enough)
- You only need to perform each exercise once. The only exceptions are noted in the exercises themselves, such as when you might change a handgrip.
- Never jerk, snap, or suddenly move your muscles. Isometrics, properly done, are all

about steadily increasing the tension, holding it, and then steadily releasing it.
- Although I do recommend that you exercise daily, you should never exercise more than once a day.
- You should never experience pain when performing these exercises. If you do feel pain, try exercising as hard as you can just short of that pain threshold. If the pain persists, however, see a doctor.
- You may find that your muscles quiver a bit when first starting out. So long as it is not painful do not let this concern you. It is merely an indication that your muscles are working hard.
- Even with the breathing routine it is possible you will feel a little faint if you are extremely out of shape. In this case try performing the point of maximum contraction at 60% to 70% of your maximum strength and hold the contraction for 12 seconds instead of 7. As your body gets used to the exercise the feeling of faintness should fade. At that point you can start to increase the intensity while decreasing the time.
- When breathing in ALWAYS breathe through your nose. There are two reasons for this. The first is that your nose is designed to breathe in air. It purifies and prepares the air you breathe to enter your delicate lungs in a way that your mouth does not. The second reason is that breathing in through your nose is relaxing for your body whereas mouth breathing sends panic signals to your brain. You will

make much faster progress if your body is relaxed as opposed to stressed.

How To Perform This Isometric Workout

The isometric routine that follows is quite simple to perform. The only wrinkle is that some of the exercises, such as the Biceps Curl, actually contain 3 positions. The reason for this is that an isometric contraction most effectively builds strength within a range of roughly 20 degrees in either direction from where it is performed. Therefore, in order to build strength for the full range of motion, it is necessary to perform the isometric contraction at three different angles. My recommendation is that when you perform this workout you adopt a 3-day cycle. So, on Day 1 you perform all of the exercises, including the position A ones where applicable. On Day 2 perform all of the exercises, except now perform Position B. On Day 3, do Position C. Rinse and repeat.

After you complete a 3-day cycle I recommend you rest on the 4th day before beginning a fresh cycle. Now, let's get to the workout itself.

Abdominal Exercises

Isometric Stomach Flattener

This exercise can be done from either the standing or sitting position. The advantage of performing it standing is that it will work the muscles in your abdomen and buttocks. The advantage of doing it sitting is that it can be done anywhere, including at work.

1. Pull your abdomen in as hard as you can as you breathe through your nose for 3 seconds. Imagine you are trying to force your abdomen against your backbone.
2. Hold this contraction as hard as you can while simultaneously breathing out through your mouth for 7 seconds. Make sure you make the "ssssssss" sound.
3. Breathe in again through your nose for 3 seconds as you relax the tension in your stomach muscles.

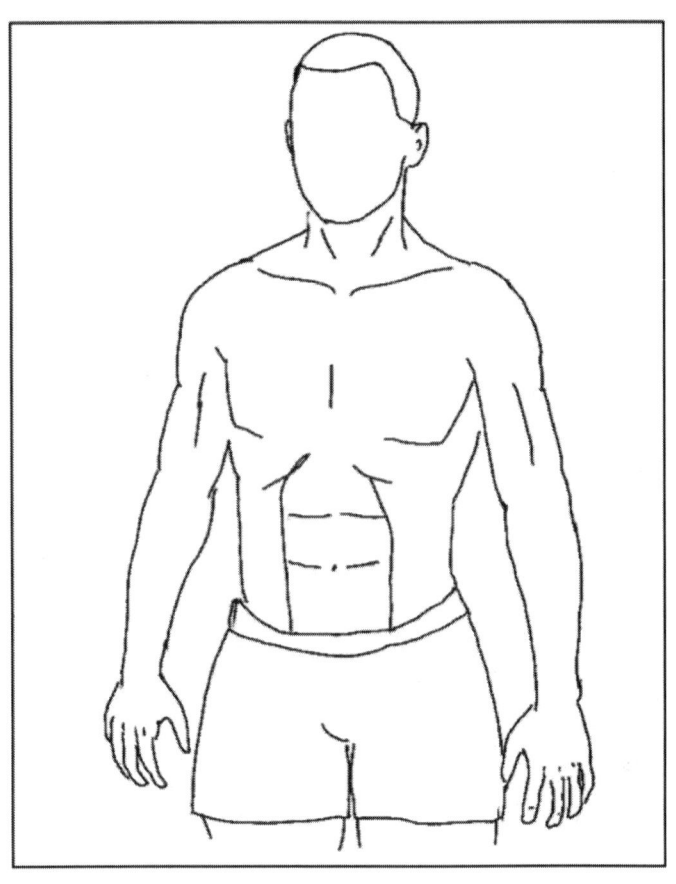

Oblique Door Press

The oblique muscles, which are on either side of your waist, help to stabilize your upper body. This exercise will ensure that these muscles stay strong.

1. Stand with your left side about 6 to 8 inches away from a wall or doorway.
2. Raise your right hand overhead and place it against the wall.
3. As you breathe in through your nose for 3 seconds, use your oblique muscles to press your hand against the wall.
4. Hold this contraction for 7 seconds as you breathe out through your mouth, making the "sssssss" sound.
5. Breathe in again through your nose for 3 seconds as you relax your muscles.

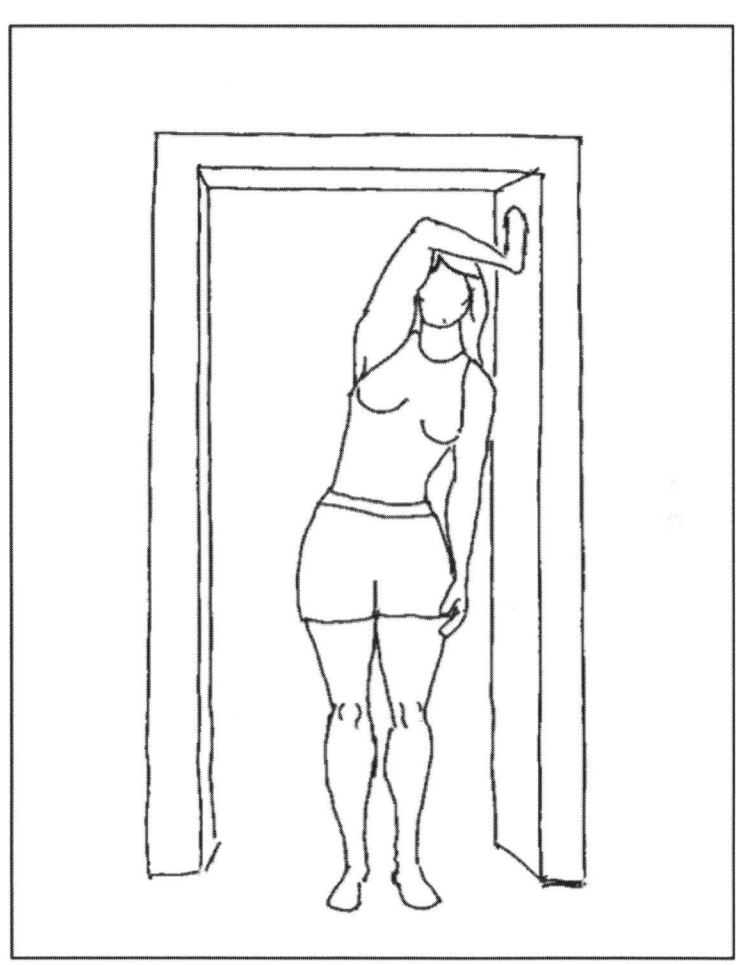

Exercises For The Neck

Reverse Neck Contraction

This isometric exercise will build up the muscles in the back of your neck. It has three positions. Position A begins with your neck bent forward and your chin tucked into your chest. Position B, which is pictured and described below, begins with the neck straight. Position C involves starting with your neck bent backwards as if you are trying to look up at the ceiling.

1. Begin with your abs contracted, your back straight, and your knees slightly bent.
2. Keeping your neck straight clasp your hands and place them behind your head.
3. Start increasing the pressure on your palms by pressing the back of your head against them for 3 seconds while you inhale through your nose.
4. Hold this contraction for 7 seconds as you breathe out through your mouth making the "ssssssss" sound.
5. Relax the pressure as you breathe in through your nose for 3 seconds.

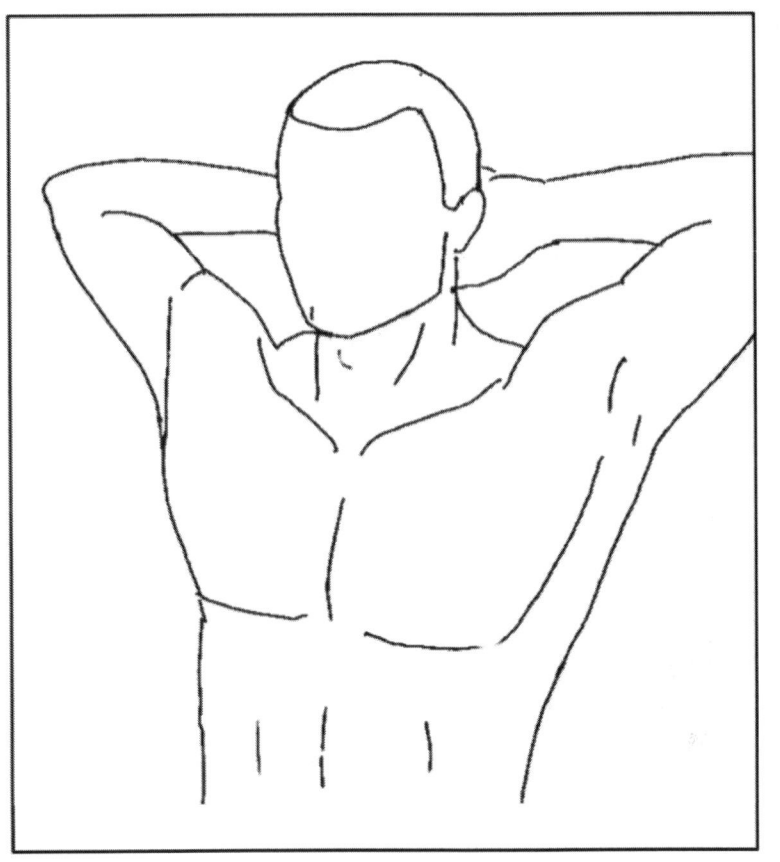

Forward Neck Contraction

This exercise uses three positions to build up muscles in the front of the neck. Position A begins with your neck bent forward so that your chin is touching your chest. With Position B, which is described and pictured below, your neck is straight. Position C begins with your neck bent backwards.

1. Begin with your abs contracted, your back straight, and your knees slightly bent.
2. Keeping your neck straight make a fist with one hand and place it on your forehead with your thumb touching it. Clasp the top of your fist with the other hand.
3. Start increasing the pressure on your fist by pressing your head forward for 3 seconds while your breathe through your nose. Remember, your head should never actually move.
4. Hold this contraction for 7 seconds as you breathe out through your mouth making the "ssssssss" sound.
5. Relax the pressure as you breathe in through your nose for 3 seconds.

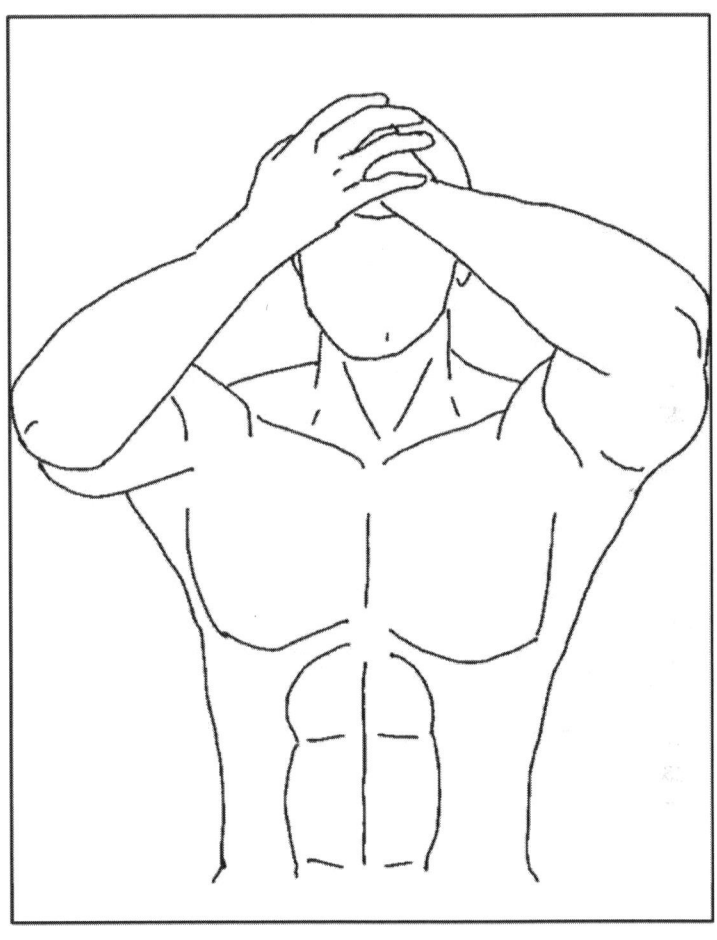

Side Neck Contraction

The three positions for this exercise will build up the muscles along the side of the neck. Position A begins with the head tilted towards the left side. Position B, which is pictured and described below, involves keeping the neck straight. With Position C the head is tilted towards the opposite shoulder.

1. Begin with your abs contracted, your back straight, and your knees slightly bent.
2. With your neck straight place your right hand on the right side of your head.
3. Start increasing the pressure on your right hand by forcing your head against it. Breathe through your nose for 3 seconds as you increase the pressure. Remember, your head should never actually move.
4. Hold this contraction for 7 seconds as you breathe out through your mouth making the "sssssss" sound.
5. Relax the pressure as you breathe in through your nose for 3 seconds.
6. Reverse and repeat this exercise for the left side of your head.

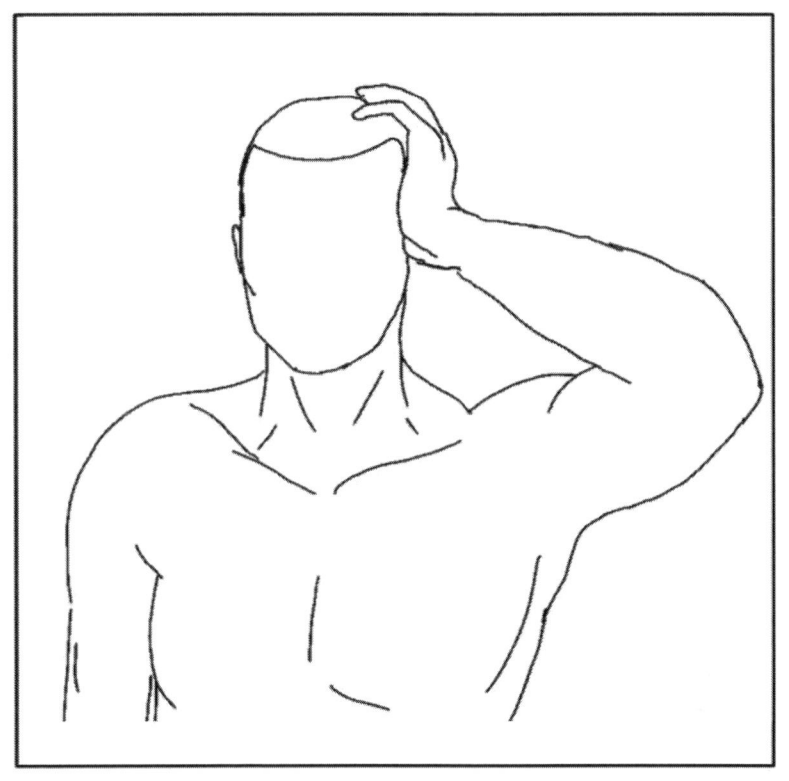

Exercises For The Back

Trapezius Contraction

1. Begin by sitting in a sturdy armless chair with your feet about 12 inches apart.
2. With your back straight and abs tight, grab the bottom of the chair.
3. Slowly begin to raise / shrug your shoulders backwards and upwards, almost as if you are trying to touch them behind your ears. Resist this upward shoulder shrug by pulling on the bottom of the chair.
4. As you breathe in through your nose for 3 seconds you should feel the tension increase in your upper back and neck.
5. Hold this contraction for 7 seconds as you breathe out through your mouth making the "ssssssss" sound.
6. Relax the tension as you breathe in through your nose for 3 seconds.

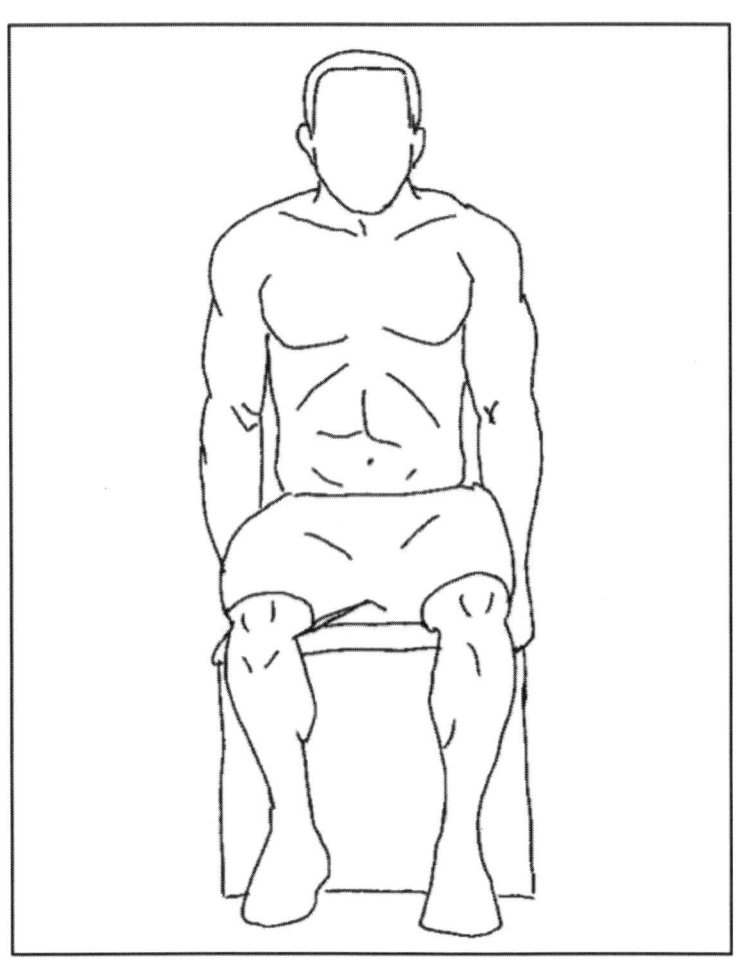

The Isometric Row

With the Isometric Row there are two positions. Position A, which is described and shown below, is performed with the arms roughly parallel with the shoulders. Position B is done with your arms sloping downward at a 45-degree angle from your trunk, allowing you to exercise the middle of the back. I usually perform both positions on the same day, although you can split them up if you wish.

1. Begin with your feet shoulder-width apart and your knees slightly bent.
2. Bring both arms straight out in front of you. Pretend as if you are grasping a broom handle with both hands.
3. Pull the imaginary broom handle backwards. It is almost as if you are attempting to touch your elbows together behind your back.
4. Breathe in through your nose for 3 seconds as you generate tension by attempting to squeeze your shoulder blades and elbows together.
5. Hold this contraction for 7 seconds as you breathe out through your mouth making the "ssssssss" sound.
6. Relax the pressure as you breathe in through your nose for 3 seconds.

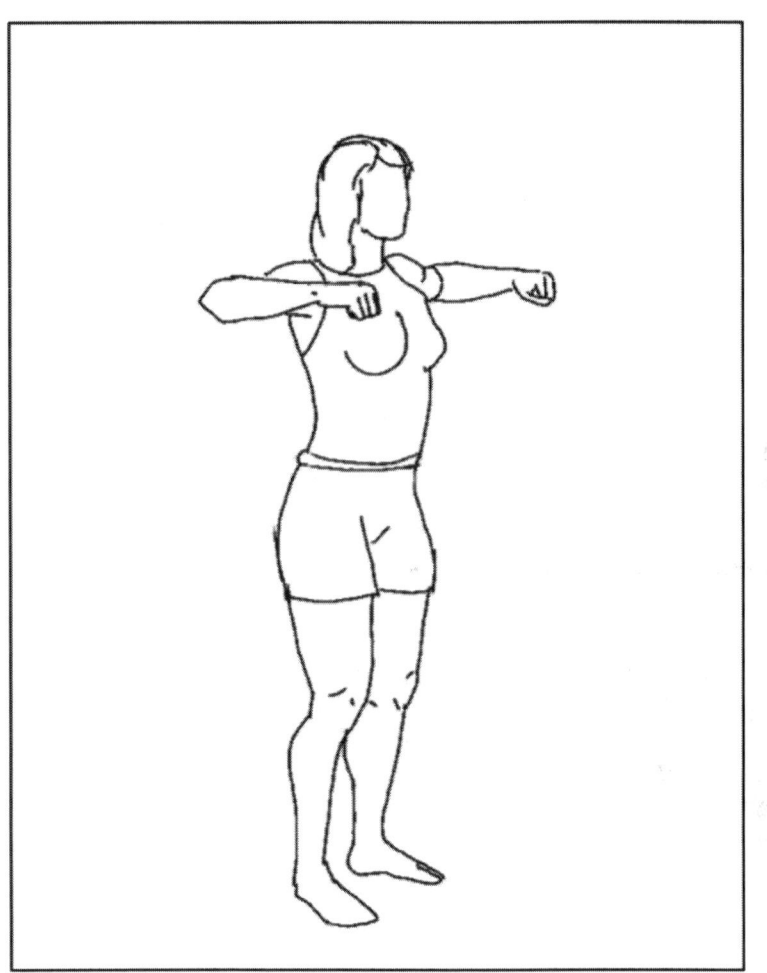

Sitting Isometric Pull

This exercise works the latissimus dorsi muscles, which are the large fanned muscles in the upper back. This exercise has 3 positions. Position A, which is shown and described below, begins with your arms straight and your foot just off the ground. With Position B you will want to raise your knee about 4 inches higher than in Position A. Position C involves beginning with your right knee close to your chest.

1. Begin by sitting in a chair with no armrests.
2. Use both hands to interlock your fingers underneath your right knee. Your arms should be straight.
3. Breathe in through your nose for 3 seconds as you use your back muscles to pull on your knee while you simultaneously resist this effort with your leg. You should feel the tension build in your back muscles on the right side.
4. Hold this contraction for 7 seconds as you breathe out through your mouth making the "ssssssss" sound.
5. Relax the pressure as you breathe in through your nose for 3 seconds.
6. Repeat this exercise utilizing your left knee.

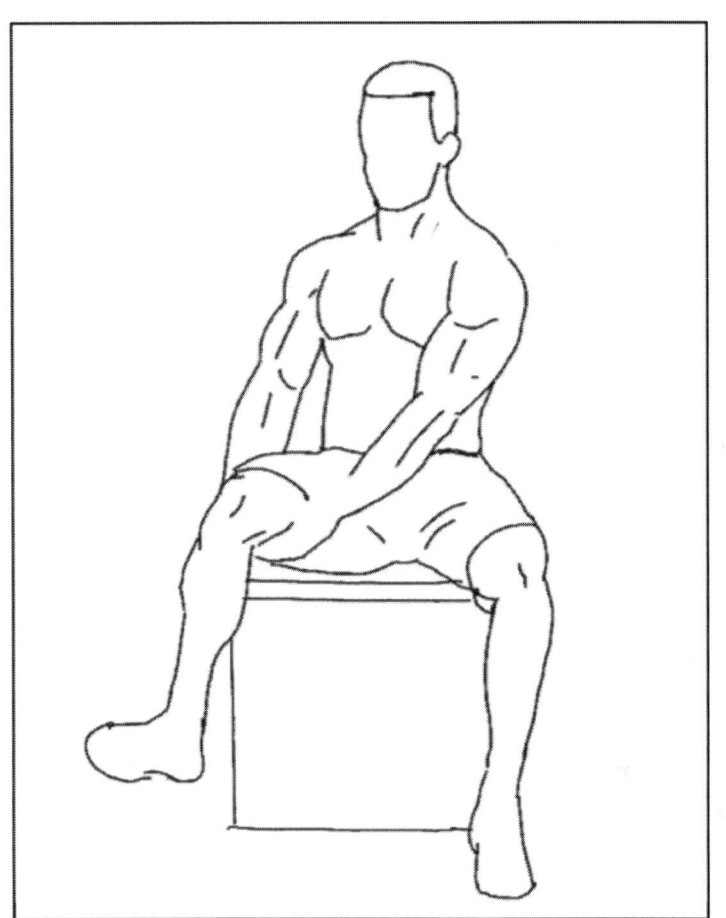

Isometric Wall Press

1. Stand facing a wall with your feet 6 to 8 inches from it.
2. Extend your arms upwards and place your palms against the wall.
3. Increase the pressure on your palms by pressing them straight ahead as you breathe in through your nose for 3 seconds.
4. Hold this contraction for 7 seconds as you breathe out through your mouth making the "sssssss" sound.
5. Relax the pressure as you breathe in through your nose for 3 seconds.

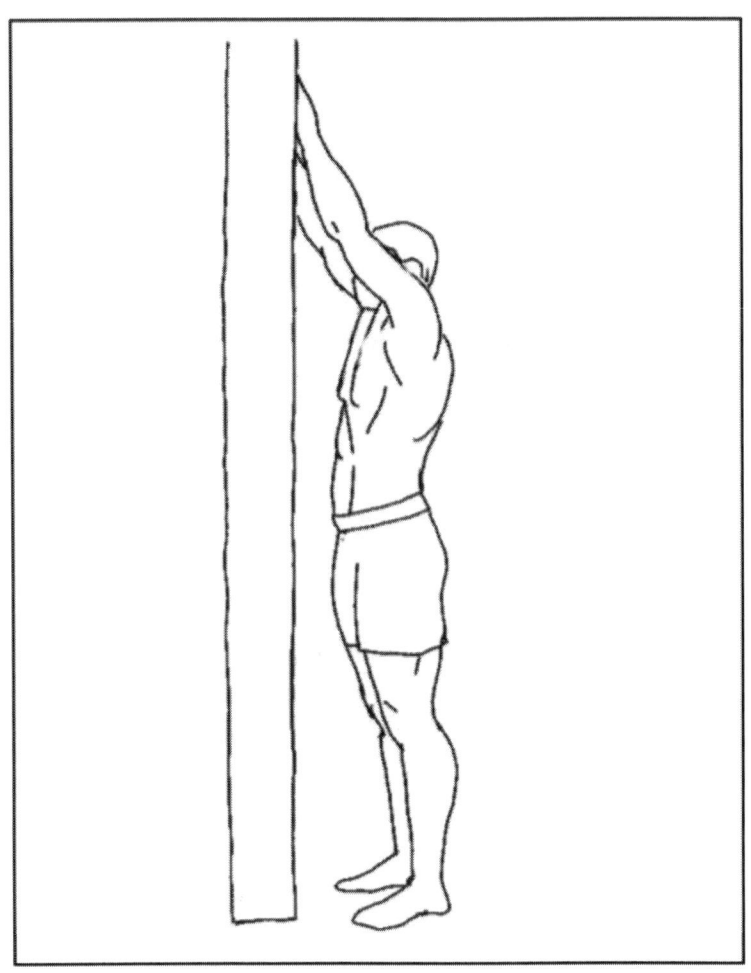

Isometric Broom Pull

1. From a semi-squatting position grasp a broom handle with your hands roughly 18 inches apart and palms facing upward.
2. Place the broom behind your knees.
3. As you breathe in through your nose for 3 seconds press the handle upward and forward against the back of your knees.
4. Hold this contraction for 7 seconds as you breathe out through your mouth making the "ssssssss" sound.
5. Breathe in through your nose for 3 seconds as you release the contraction.
6. Make sure you keep your back straight during the entire exercise.

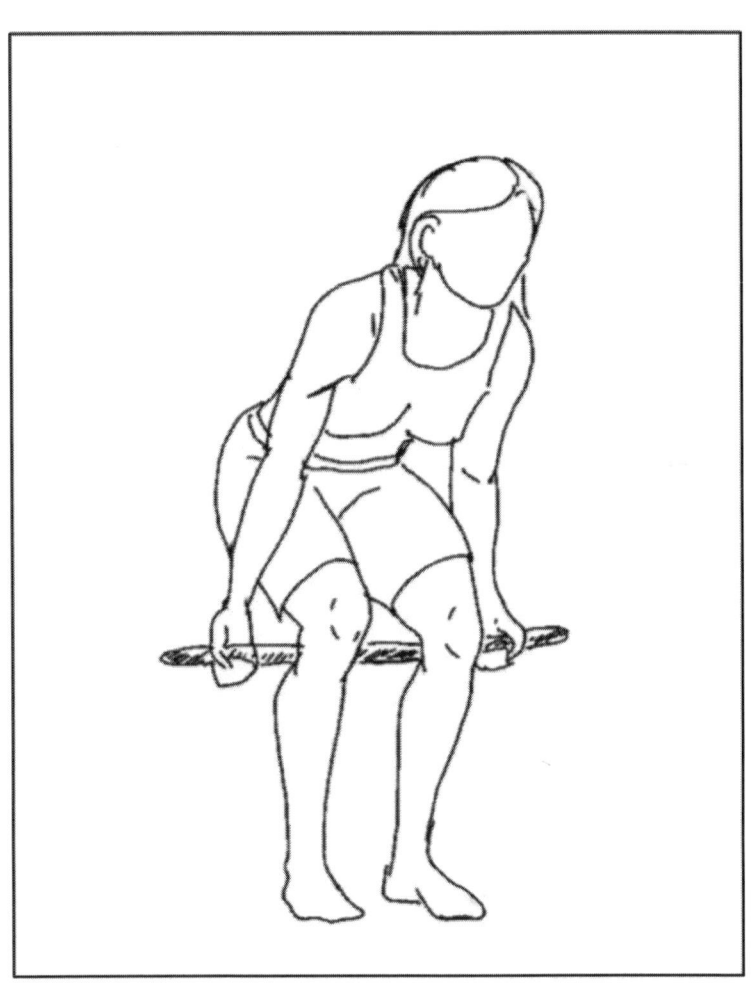

The Isometric Superman

1. Lie face down on the floor with your arms stretched out like you're superman.
2. As you breathe in through your nose for 3 seconds use your back muscles to lift your chest off the ground. Your feet should remain in contact with the ground at all times.
3. Hold this contraction for 7 seconds as you breathe out through your mouth making the "ssssssss" sound.
4. Breathe in through your nose for 3 seconds as you relax your back muscles while lowering your chest to the ground.

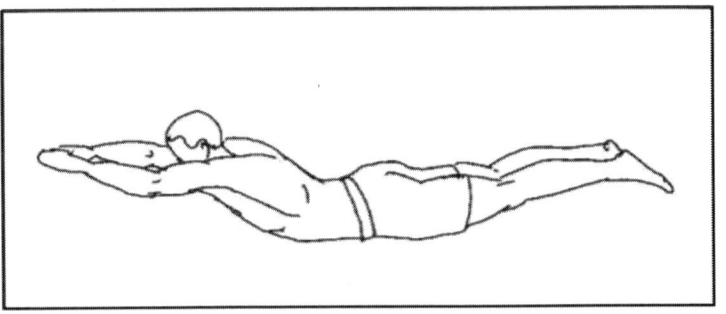

Shoulder Exercises

Isometric Shoulder Press

The exercise has three positions. With Position A you will want to begin with your fist so that it is inline with your shoulder. For Position B, which is pictured and described below, begin with your fist inline with your forehead. Position C is performed with your fist raised just above your head.

1. Begin with your back straight and your feet shoulder width apart.
2. Bend your right elbow so that your clenched right fist is inline with your forehead.
3. Place your left hand over your right fist.
4. Begin to press your right fist upwards while you breathe in through your nose for 3 seconds. Resist this motion with your left hand. Remember that your arm should never move.
5. Hold this contraction for 7 seconds as you breathe out through your mouth making the "sssssss" sound.
6. Breathe in through your nose for 3 seconds as you relax your muscles.
7. Repeat this exercise by placing your right hand over your left fist.

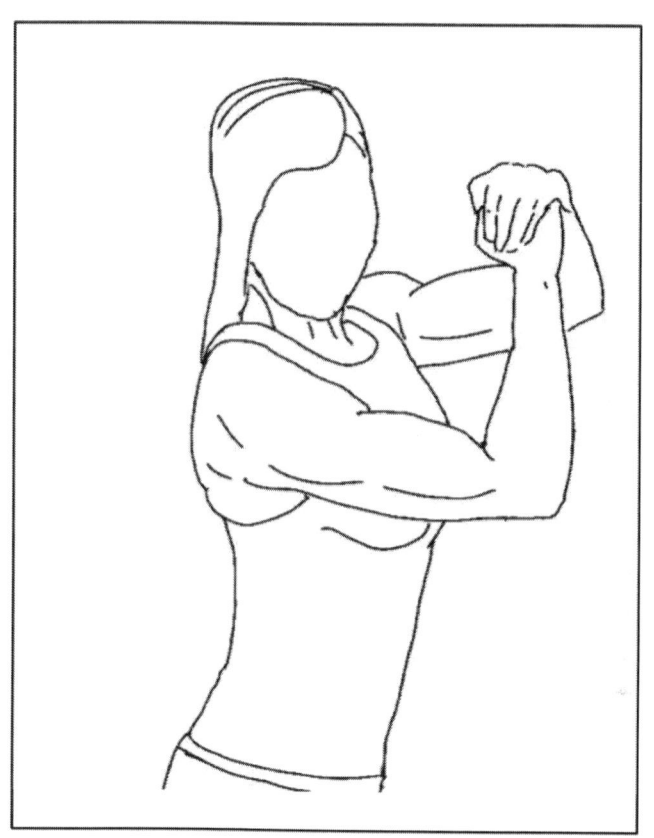

Front Shoulder Raise

This exercise works the front of the shoulder. It contains three positions. Position A is performed with your fist about 6 inches above your thigh. Position B, which is described and pictured below, is done with your arm at a 45-degree angle from your body. Position C is performed with your arm positioned at a 90-degree angle from your body, your fist at or just above your shoulders.

1. Begin with your feet shoulder width apart and your knees slightly bent.
2. Clench your right fist as tightly as possible while positioning your arm at a 45-degree angle in front of your body. Your right elbow should have a slight bend to it as opposed to being completely locked out.
3. Place your left hand over your right fist.
4. Begin to breathe in through your nose for 3 seconds as you attempt to use your shoulder to raise your right arm while resisting with your left hand. Remember that your arm should never move.
5. Hold this contraction for 7 seconds as you breathe out through your mouth making the "ssssssss" sound.
6. Breathe in through your nose for 3 seconds as you relax your muscles.
7. Repeat this exercise with the opposite arm.

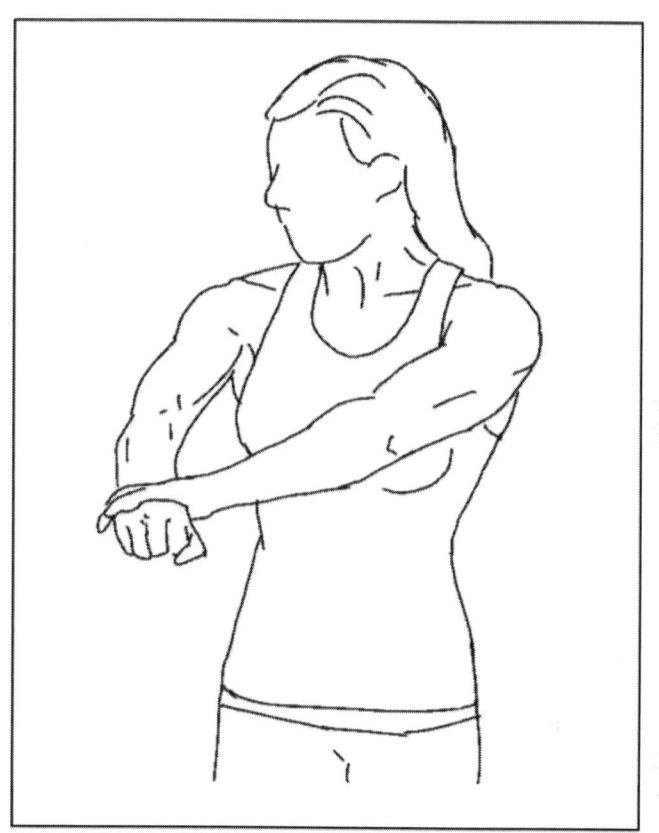

Side Shoulder Raise

This exercise works the side of the shoulder. It contains three positions. Position A is performed with your arm at a 6-degree angle from your body. Position B, which is described and pictured below, begins with your arm at a 45-degree angle from your body. Position C is performed with your arm positioned at a 90-degree angle from your shoulders.

1. Begin with your feet shoulder width apart and your knees slightly bent.
2. Clench your right fist as tightly as possible while positioning your arm at a 45-degree angle from the side of your body and your right elbow bent.
3. Place your left hand over your right fist.
4. Begin to breathe in through your nose for 3 seconds as you attempt to use your shoulder to raise your right arm while resisting with your left hand. Remember that your arm should never move.
5. Hold this contraction for 7 seconds as you breathe out through your mouth making the "ssssssss" sound.
6. Breathe in through your nose for 3 seconds as you relax your muscles.
7. Repeat this exercise with the opposite arm.

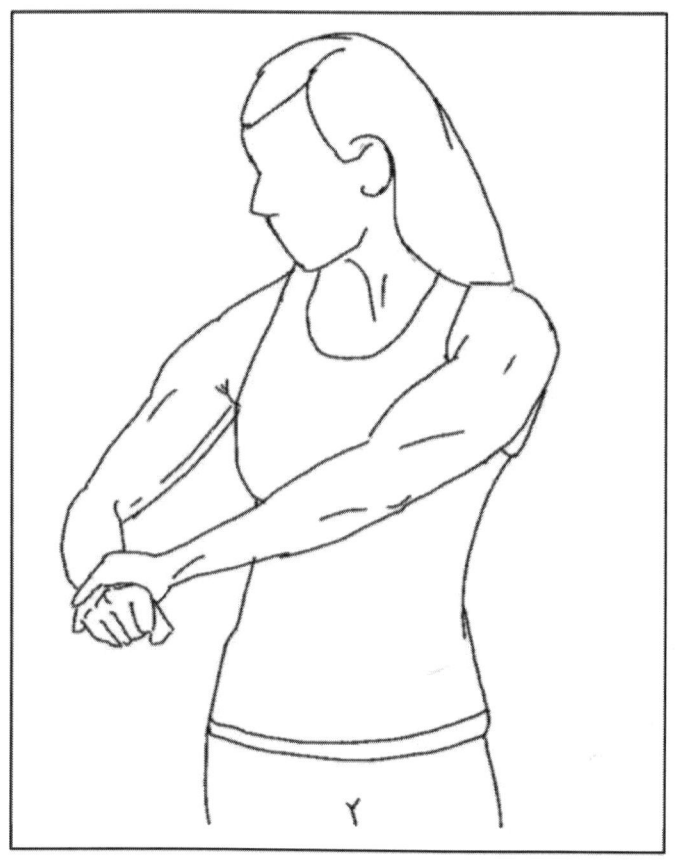

٢

Rear Shoulder Pull

This exercise will work the back of your shoulders. To work these muscles you will be preventing your arm from coming towards you, as opposed to raising it away from your body. There are three positions for this exercise. Position A begins with your arm 6 inches from the center of your body. Position B, which is described and pictured below, begins with your arm at a 45-degree angle. Position C is done with your arm at a 90-degree angle from the center of your body.

1. Begin with your feet shoulder width apart and your knees slightly bent.
2. Clench your right fist as tightly as possible while positioning your arm at a 45-degree angle from the front of your body. Your fist should be roughly in the center of your body.
3. Use your left hand to grab the top of your right wrist.
4. Begin to breathe in through your nose for 3 seconds as you attempt to use your back shoulder muscles to lower your right arm towards you. Your left hand will resist this motion. Remember that your arm should never move.
5. Hold this contraction for 7 seconds as you breathe out through your mouth making the "ssssssss" sound.
6. Breathe in through your nose for 3 seconds as you relax your muscles.
7. Repeat this exercise with the opposite arm.

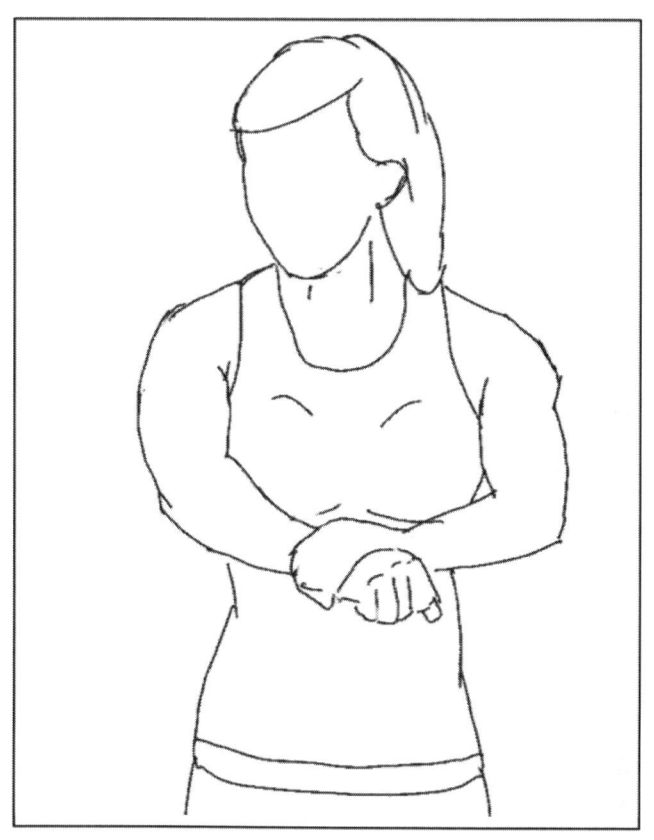

Isometric Arm Exercises

Biceps Curl

This exercise works the two bundles of muscles in your upper arms, otherwise known as the biceps. There are three positions for the biceps curl. Position A is performed with only a slight bend in your elbow. Position B, which is pictured and described below, is done with your elbow at a 90-degree angle. Position C is performed with your fist almost parallel to your shoulder.

1. Begin with your feet shoulder width apart and your knees slightly bent.
2. Clench your right fist as tightly as possible while bending your right elbow so that an angle of 90-degrees is created between your upper and lower arm. Your upper arm should be parallel with your body while your lower arm is perpendicular to it.
3. Place your left hand over your right wrist.
4. Begin to breathe in through your nose for 3 seconds as you attempt to curl your right arm upwards, resisting with your left hand. Remember that your arm should never move.
5. Hold this contraction for 7 seconds as you breathe out through your mouth making the "sssssss" sound.
6. Breathe in through your nose for 3 seconds as you relax your arm muscles.

7. Repeat this exercise with the opposite arm.

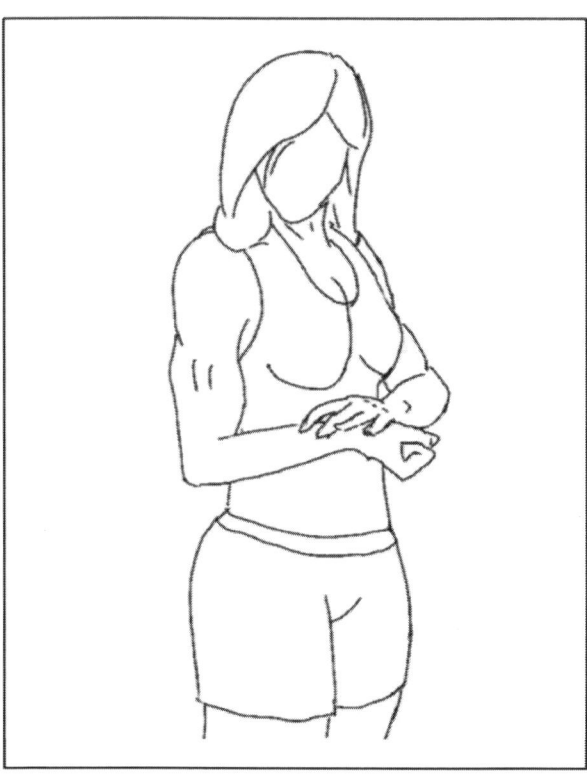

Triceps Press Down

This exercise works the three bundles of muscles located on the back of your arm. It has three positions. Position A begins with your fist almost parallel to your shoulder. Position B, pictured and described below, is performed with your elbow at a 90 degree angle. With Position C there is only a slight bend to your elbow.

1. Begin with your feet shoulder width apart and your knees slightly bent.
2. Clench your right hand into a hammer fist while bending your right elbow so that an angle of 90-degrees is created between your upper and lower arm. Your upper arm should be parallel with your body while your lower arm is perpendicular to it.
3. Place your left hand under your right fist.
4. Begin to breathe in through your nose for 3 seconds as you attempt to press your right fist downwards, resisting with your left hand. Remember that your arm should never move.
5. Hold this contraction for 7 seconds as you breathe out through your mouth making the "sssssss" sound.
6. Breathe in through your nose for 3 seconds as you relax your arm muscles.
7. Repeat this exercise with the opposite arm.

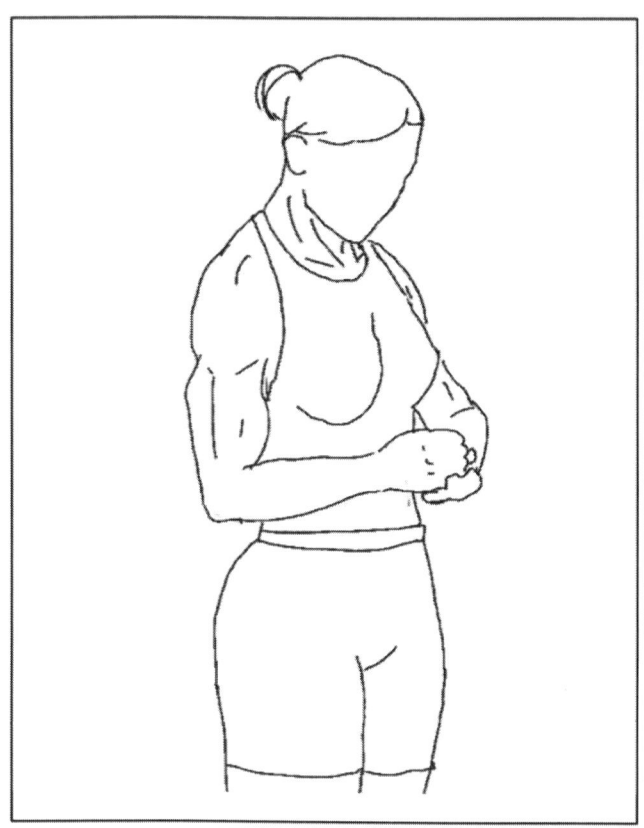

Isometric Cross Arm Contraction

This exercise works both the biceps and triceps at the same time and is made up of 3 positions. Position A is performed with your fists almost parallel with your shoulders. Position B, which is described and pictured below, is done with your fists in the middle of your chest. Position C is performed with your fists at waist level.

1. Begin with your feet shoulder width apart and your knees slightly bent.
2. Clench both of your hands into hammer fists and then place your left fist over your right in the center of your body.
3. Begin to breathe in through your nose for 3 seconds as you attempt to press your left fist downwards, resisting with your right. Remember that neither arm should ever move.
4. Hold this contraction for 7 seconds as you breathe out through your mouth making the "ssssssss" sound.
5. Breathe in through your nose for 3 seconds as you relax your arm muscles.
6. Repeat this exercise by reversing your fists.

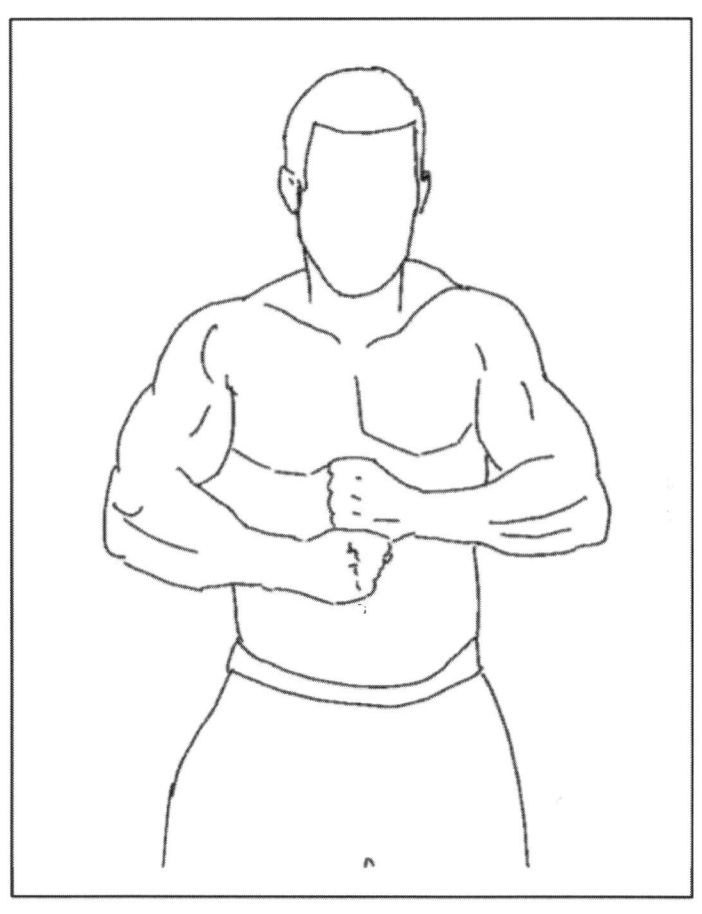

Chest Exercises

Isometric Pec Builder (Push)

This exercise has 3 potential starting points. Position A involves pressing your hands together at your stomach level. Position B is performed at chest level and is pictured and described below. Position C involves pressing your hands together just above your forehead. These three positions insure that you will be able to work your entire chest from top to bottom.

1. Press both your hands together in front of your chest.
2. Inhale through your nose for 3 seconds as you press your hands together.
3. Hold this contraction for 7 seconds as you breathe out through your mouth making the "sssssss" sound.
4. Inhale through your nose for 3 seconds as you release the pressure between your hands.
5. Repeat the exercise with the handgrip reversed.

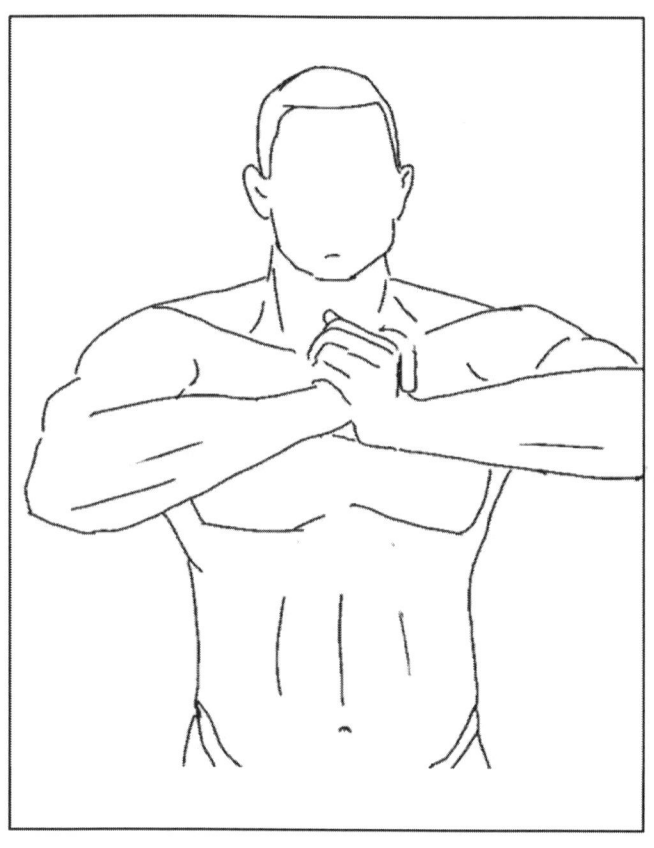

Isometric Pec Builder (Pull)

This exercise has 3 potential starting points. Position A involves pulling your hands apart at your stomach level. Position B is performed at chest level and is pictured and described below. Position C involves pulling your hands apart just above your forehead. These three positions ensure that you will be able to work your entire chest from top to bottom.

1. Clasp your hands together at chest level by intertwining your fingers like they are hooks.
2. Inhale through your nose for 3 seconds as you attempt to pull your fingers apart.
3. Hold this contraction for 7 seconds as you breathe out through your mouth making the "sssssss" sound.
4. Inhale through your nose for 3 seconds as you release the pressure between your hands.
5. Repeat the exercise with your handgrip reversed.

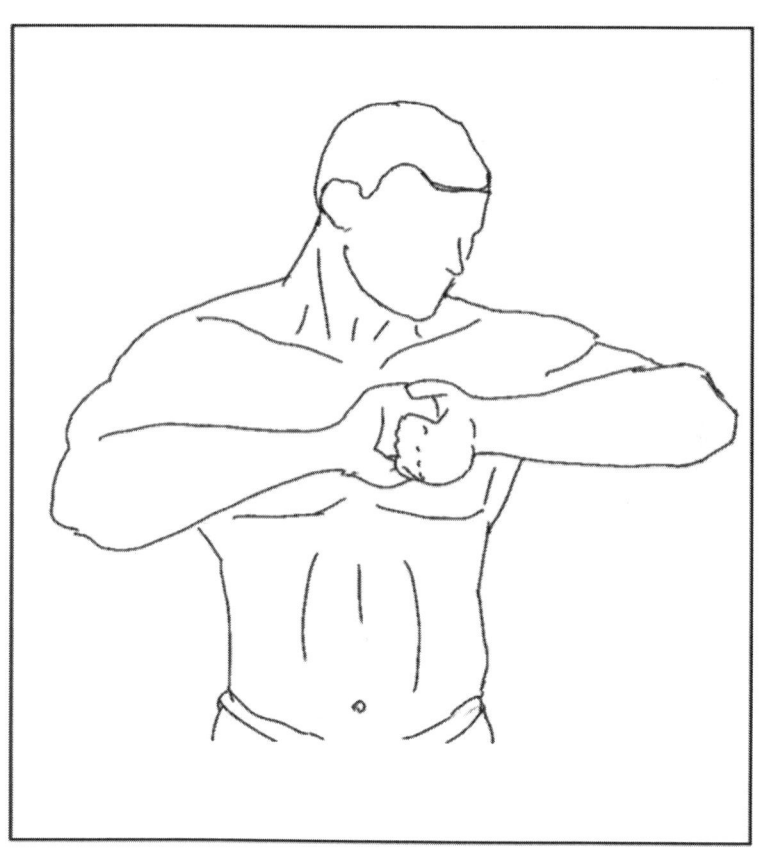

Isometric Pushup

1. Lie on the floor face down.
2. Extend your arms straight out to the sides, palms facing down.
3. Inhale through your nose for 3 seconds as you press downwards on the floor with your palms.
4. Hold this contraction for 7 seconds as you breathe out through your mouth making the "ssssssss" sound.
5. Inhale through your nose for 3 seconds as you release the pressure from your hands.

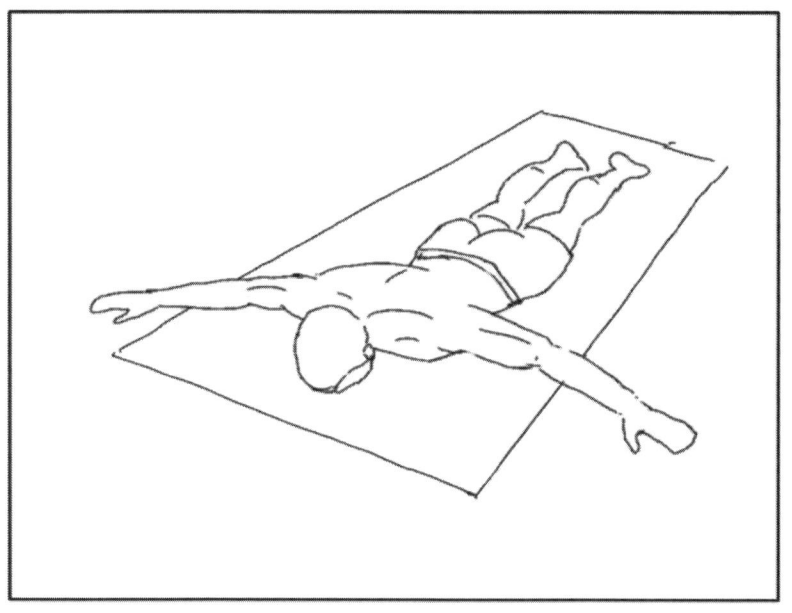

Leg Exercises

Wall Squat

There are three positions for this exercise. Position A, which is pictured and described below, involves keeping the feet flat on the floor. Position B is exactly the same, except this time you will want to raise your toes off the ground. Position C is performed by raising your heels off the ground so that you are on your tiptoes.

1. Perform a half squat with your back against a solid wall. You will want your knees to be at a 90-degree angle. If you can't get your knees to this angle, just lower your body as much as you can.
2. Inhale through your nose for 3 seconds as you press your back and butt against the wall. Imagine you are trying to push the wall over by pressing your back against it.
3. Hold this contraction for 7 seconds as you breathe out through your mouth making the "sssssss" sound.
4. Inhale through your nose for 3 seconds as you release the pressure from your back.

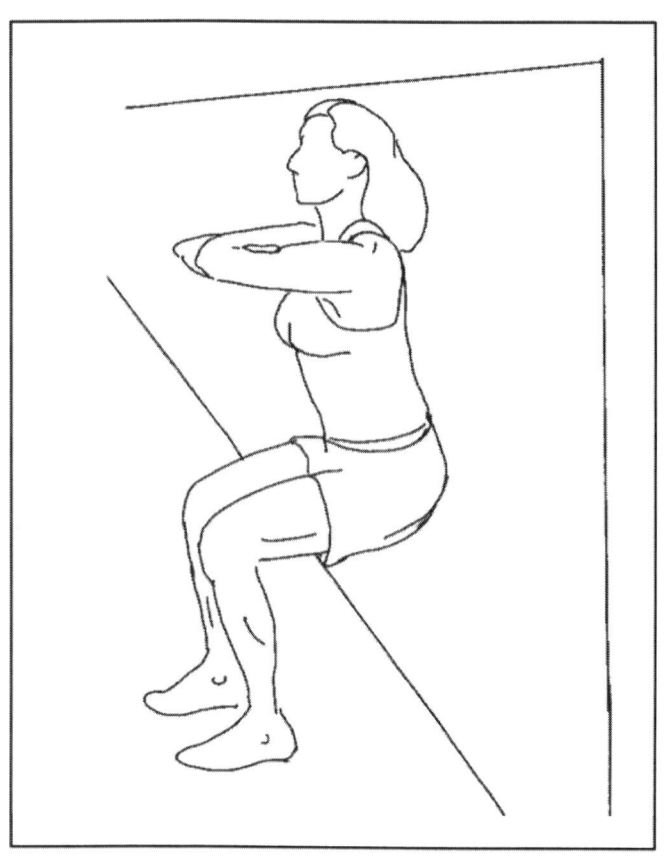

Leg Curl

There are three positions associated with the leg curl. With Position A, which is described and pictured below, your feet should be 3 inches off the ground. Position B involves raising your feet 6 inches off the ground. With Position C your knees should be bent at a 90-degree angle.

1. Lie face down on a flat surface with your head raised slightly. If you find it more comfortable you can rest your head on your hands and shoulders.
2. Wrap your left foot around your right ankle and raise your feet 3 inches off the ground.
3. Inhale through your nose for 3 seconds as you attempt to raise your right foot while resisting with your left. You should only feel an increase in tension between your feet. Your legs should never actually move.
4. Hold this contraction for 7 seconds as you breathe out through your mouth making the "sssssss" sound.
5. Inhale through your nose for 3 seconds as you release the pressure from your feet.
6. Repeat this exercise by wrapping your right foot around your left.

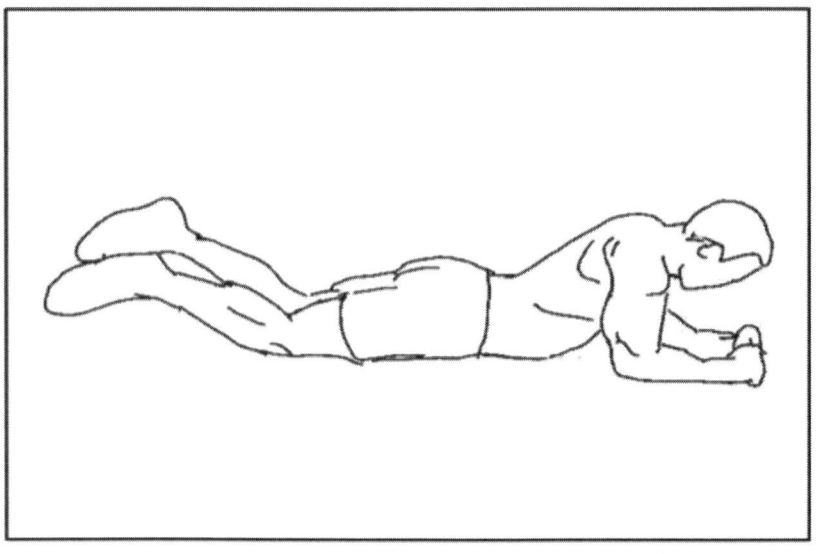

Front Thigh Exercise

There are three positions associated with this exercise. Position A, pictured and described below, involves raising your feet a few inches off the ground. With Position B you will want to raise your feet 6 inches off the ground. Position C involves straightening your legs as much as possible so that your knee is barely bent.

1. Sit in a chair. An armless chair is preferred as this will allow you to grasp the side of the seat with your hands.
2. With your legs close together place your left ankle over the front of your right foot.
3. Inhale through your nose for 3 seconds as you attempt to raise your right foot while resisting with your left. You should only feel an increase in tension between your feet, your legs should never actually move.
4. Hold this contraction for 7 seconds as you breathe out through your mouth making the "sssssss" sound.
5. Inhale through your nose for 3 seconds as you release the pressure from your feet.
6. Repeat this exercise by placing your right ankle over the front of your left foot.

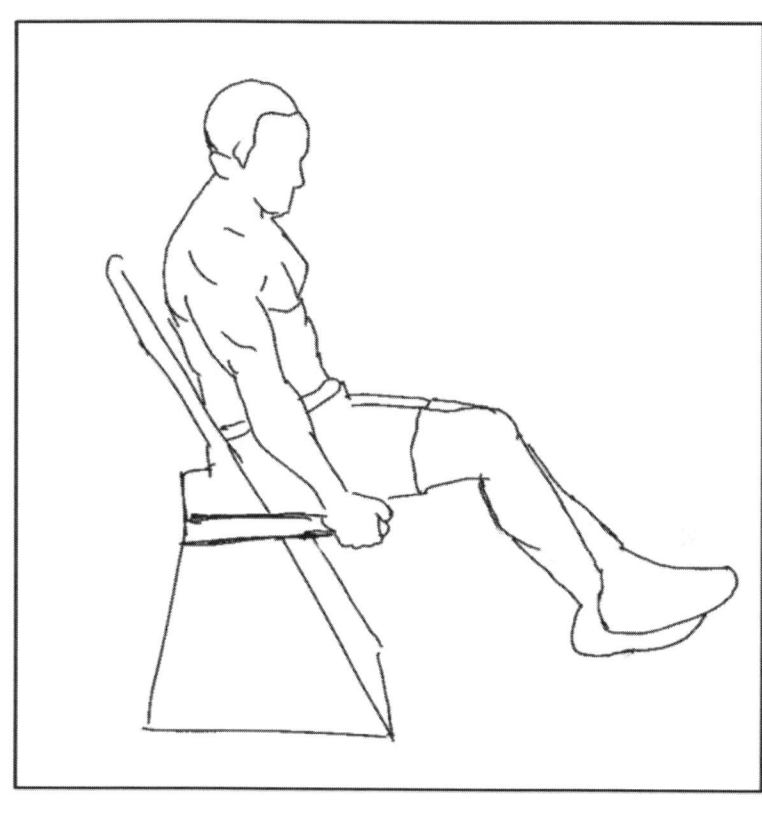

Inner Thigh Exercise

1. Sit in a chair with your feet 12 inches apart.
2. Place the palms of each hand on the knee opposite to it (right to left and left to right).
3. Breathe in through your nose for 3 seconds as you begin to try and close your thighs, resisting this motion with your hands.
4. Hold the point of maximum tension for 7 seconds while breathing out, making a "ssssssss" sound.
5. Slowly relax the tension in your legs while breathing in through your nose for another 3 seconds.

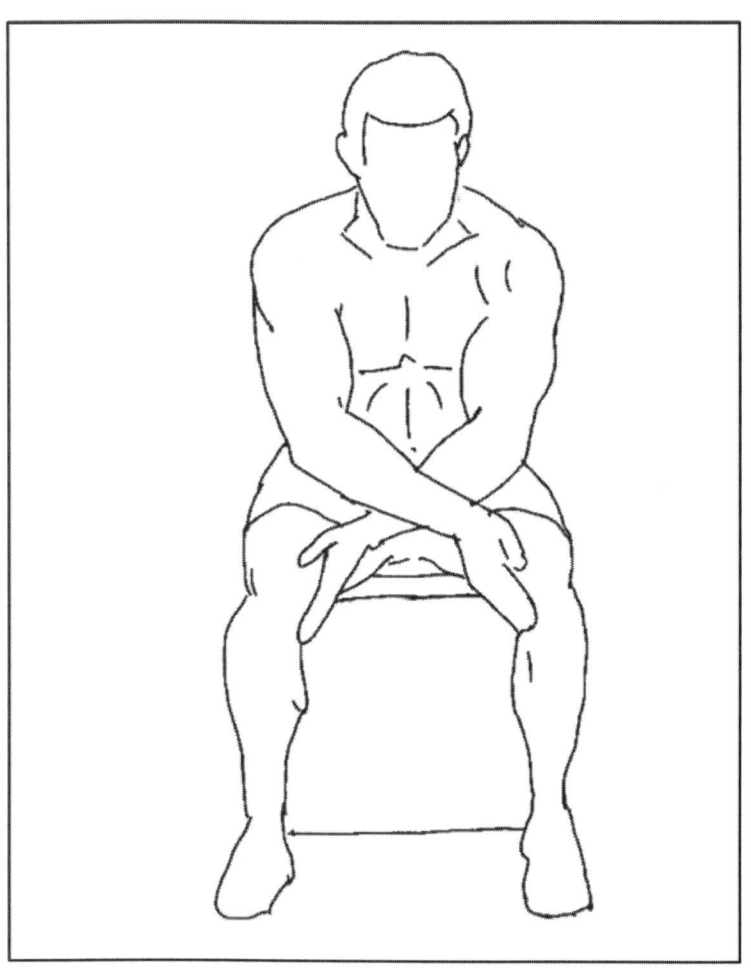

Outer Thigh Exercise

1. Sit in an armless chair with your feet 12 inches apart.
2. Place the palms of your hands on the outside of each knee.
3. Inhale through your nose for 3 seconds as you attempt to widen your thighs, resisting this motion with your hands. Your legs should never actually move.
4. Hold this contraction for 7 seconds as you breathe out through your mouth making the "ssssssss" sound.
5. Inhale through your nose for 3 seconds as you relax your legs.

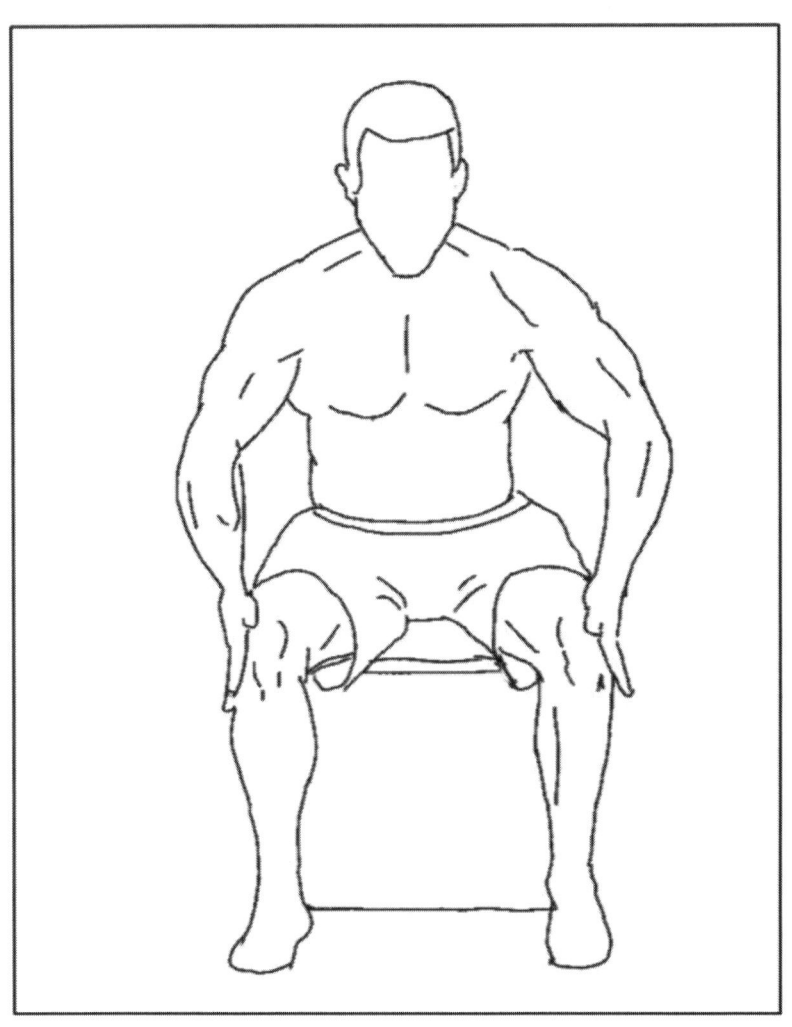

The Isometric Atlas

In Greek myth Atlas supported the entire weight of the world on his shoulders. In this exercise you will do something similar. The Isometric Atlas not only works your legs, but your entire body and is a great way to end your isometric workout.

1. Stand in a doorway or an area that contains a low, solid ceiling or similar structure. It needs to be low enough so that you can place your palms on it with your arms slightly bent.
2. Keeping your abs tight and your back straight place the palms of your hands on the surface above your head. Ideally both your legs and arms should be slightly bent.
3. Inhale through your nose for 3 seconds as you attempt to press down with your legs while pressing up with your arms. Keep your back straight and abs tight at all times.
4. Hold this contraction for 7 seconds as you breathe out through your mouth making the "sssssss" sound.
5. Inhale through your nose for 3 seconds as you relax your body.

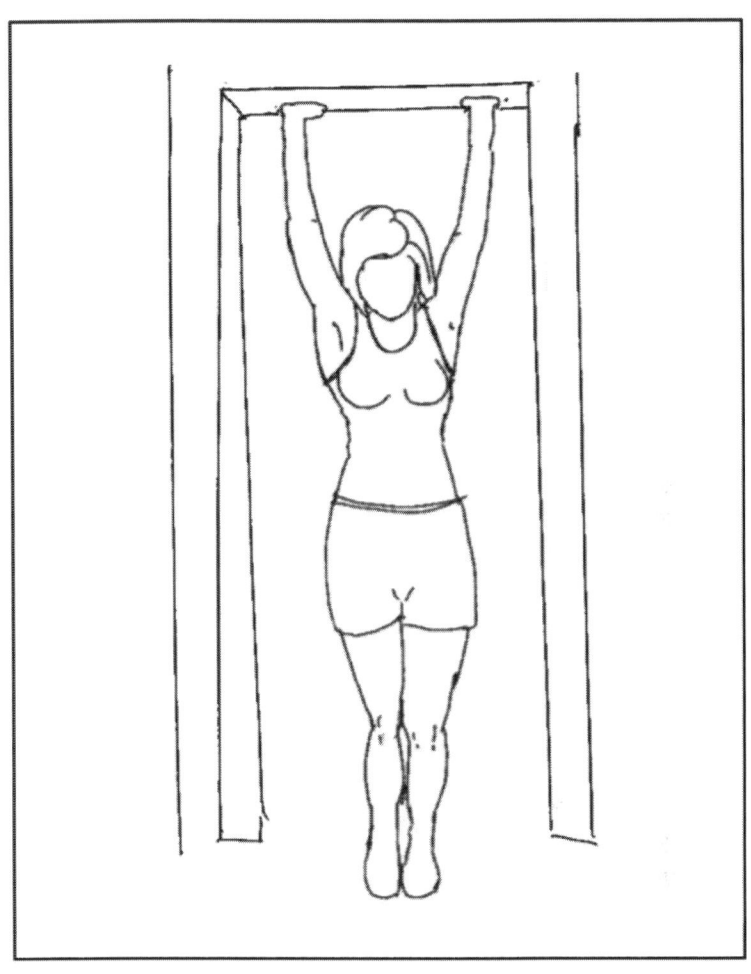

About The Author

Anthony Anholt has been interested and involved in athletics and fitness for his entire life. His specialty is "gym less" workouts, or exercise systems that do not require any kind of special equipment. He is also interested in enhancing performance in all sports, but particularly basketball.

One Last Thing

When you turn the page, Kindle will give you the opportunity to rate the book and share your thoughts through an automatic feed to your Facebook and Twitter accounts. If you believe your friends would get something valuable out of this book, I'd be honored if you'd post your thoughts. As well, if you liked the book, I'd be eternally grateful if you posted a review on Amazon. Thank-you once again and I hope you enjoyed the book!

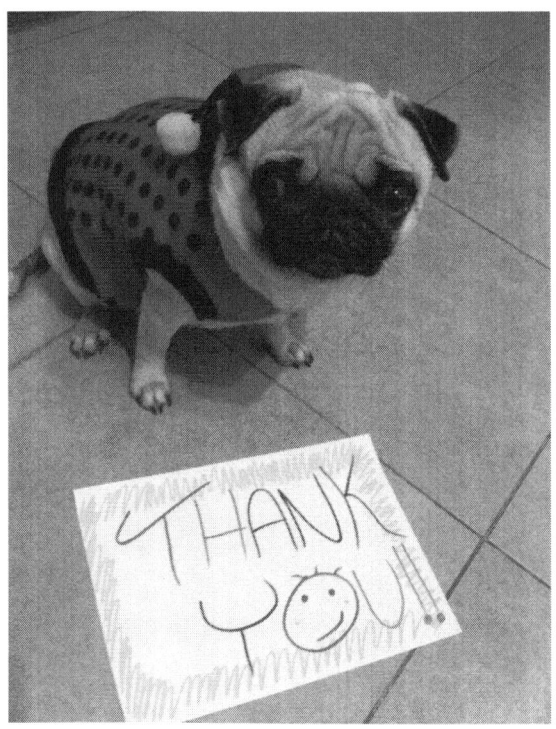

Made in the USA
San Bernardino, CA
19 September 2014